The Sweet Solution:

Your Guide to a Healthier, Energized Life

By

Berta P. Nicholls

Copyright © by **Berta P. Nicholls 2023. All rights reserved.**

TABLE OF CONTENTS

Introduction

In the flow of life, amidst the various difficulties of health and energy, one important tune orchestrates the music of our well-being – blood sugar balance. Just as a master carefully leads an orchestra, our bodies synchronize through the delicate balancing of blood sugar levels, shaping the course of our health.

In this fascinating trip, we dive deep into the world of blood sugar, discovering its vast importance and the changing potential it holds. Like a guide leading us through unknown territory, we'll explore the environment of uneven blood sugar, knowing its far-reaching effects on our energy and endurance.

Imagine blood sugar as the thread connecting the complex bits of our body processes – from energy production to mood regulation, and even the prevention of chronic diseases. Yet, the modern lifestyle often leads us wrong, causing this important thread to break and unwind. Imbalanced blood sugar, a result of our food choices and daily habits, can cast shadows on our well-being, adding to several health issues.

The Sweet Solution

But amid this setting of difficulties comes a light of hope – the promise of " The Sweet Solution." Embarking on this trip, we surpass the limits of conventional thought, accepting a new method that allows us to reclaim control over our health. The Sweet Solution is more than an idea; it's a changing road to permanent health.

As we set forth on this journey, we will uncover the science behind blood sugar, explain its complex dance with insulin and glucagon, and reveal the effects of mismatches. Together, we'll discover the secret villains in our meals, and learn the art of creating balanced plates that feed and support us. We'll discover the deep effect of physical exercise, stress management, and sleep on blood sugar balance, and how we can combine these practices into our lives.

The Sweet Solution isn't just about facts and figures; it's a story of strength, a call to action to build a personalized blood sugar control plan that fits our unique rhythms and tastes. It's about adopting a lifestyle that fills us with energy, resiliency, and the hope of a healthy future.

So, join us on this musical trip. Let's turn the page and dive into the chapters that await, as we explore the art of balancing our health through the changing power of balanced blood sugar – the Sweet Journey to Wellness.

Chapter 1: The Science of Blood Sugar

In the complicated orchestra of human physiology, the symphony of health starts with the rhythm of blood sugar management. Like a well tuned conductor, our bodies precisely adjust blood sugar levels to preserve our vitality and well-being. In this chapter, we'll investigate the basic parts of this process, exposing the astonishing function of insulin, the repercussions of insulin resistance, and the effect of rising blood sugar on our bodies. Additionally, we'll disclose the mysteries of the Glycemic Index, throwing light on the truth about carbs and their impact on blood sugar balance.

The Basics of Blood Sugar Regulation

Picture your body as a beautifully efficient mechanism, continuously seeking for equilibrium. Blood sugar, or glucose, serves as the major energy source for our cells, fueling everything from the beat of our hearts to the firing of neurons in our brains. But this valuable fuel must be kept within a tight range for optimum operation. Discover how the body manages blood sugar levels, creating a complex ballet to keep us running at our best.

The Role of Insulin in Your Body

Meet insulin, the main actor in the blood sugar symphony. Produced by the pancreas, insulin functions as a messenger, moving glucose from our circulation into our cells, where it may be utilized for energy. Explore the sophisticated processes underlying insulin's functions, and grasp how this hormone is vital for maintaining stable blood sugar levels.

Causes of Insulin Resistance

Yet, there may be disharmony in this harmonic arrangement. Insulin resistance, a disease in which our cells become less receptive to the effects of insulin, may break the equilibrium. Uncover the reasons that lead to insulin resistance, from genetic predispositions to lifestyle decisions, and understand how this disease may set the scene for a number of health complications.

How High Blood Sugar Harms Your Body

The implications of elevated blood sugar extend well beyond a transient energy boost. Persistent high levels might wreak havoc on our health. From cardiovascular issues to neurological damage, the effect is substantial. Discover the complicated network of physiological changes induced by unregulated blood sugar, providing light on why it's necessary to keep this critical parameter in balance.

The Glycemic Index: Unveiling the Truth about Carbohydrates

Not all carbs are created equal, and the Glycemic Index (GI) holds the key to understanding this disparity. Delve into the notion of the GI, a vital instrument that assesses how rapidly various meals boost blood sugar levels. Explore the consequences of high and low GI foods, and discover how to make educated dietary choices that support stable blood sugar and general well-being.

As we continue on this scientific adventure, remember that knowing the science of blood sugar is the basis for the transforming journey ahead.

By mastering these basic principles, we empower ourselves to make educated decisions, setting the scene for the Sugar Shift that lies ahead.

Chapter 2: The Sugar Rollercoaster

In the delicate area of blood sugar management, there exists a phenomenon that parallels the excitement and unpredictability of a rollercoaster ride — the Sugar Rollercoaster. This chapter uncovers the physiological subtleties of this trip, addressing the peaks and valleys of blood sugar surges, their consequences on our well-being, and techniques to negotiate the ride with grace.

The Highs and Lows of Blood Sugar Spikes

Imagine indulging in a carbohydrate-rich dinner — your favorite pasta dish, say, or a sweet dessert. As you relish each mouthful, your body goes into action, breaking down carbs into glucose, which enters the circulation. This burst of glucose generates a quick increase in blood sugar levels, resulting to what's frequently referred to as a "blood sugar spike." This is the exciting ascension of the Sugar Rollercoaster.

However, what goes up must ultimately come down. The body reacts to these high blood sugar levels by generating insulin, a hormone that transports glucose into cells for energy or storage.

This mechanism helps decrease blood sugar, but it might overshoot, leading to an abrupt drop in blood sugar levels — the crash of the Sugar Rollercoaster. This crash is marked by exhaustion, irritability, shakiness, and acute desires for sugary or carbohydrate-rich meals to fast restore energy levels again.

How to Lower a Glucose Spike After a Meal

While the Sugar Rollercoaster may seem unavoidable, there are practical techniques to smooth its path. One crucial technique is to concentrate on the content of your meals. Incorporating a mix of complex carbs, protein, and healthy fats helps slow down the absorption of glucose, minimizing fast surges. Portion management is also crucial, since bigger meals may overwhelm the body's insulin response, leading to more dramatic oscillations.

Another important practice is mindful eating. Savoring each mouthful and eating slowly assists your body to better handle the intake of glucose, reducing unexpected spikes. Additionally, incorporating fiber-rich meals helps further regulate blood sugar levels, since fiber slows down digestion and the absorption of glucose.

The Immediate and Long-Term Effects on Your Body
Beyond the acute unpleasantness of the highs and lows, the Sugar Rollercoaster may wreak havoc on your health in the long term. Frequent and large blood sugar increases may lead to insulin resistance, a disease where your cells become less sensitive to insulin's signals, resulting in chronically increased blood sugar levels. This, in turn, lays the foundation for weight gain, higher body fat, and heightened risk of type 2 diabetes.

Furthermore, the cardiovascular system takes a blow, since elevated blood sugar may damage blood vessels and raise the risk of heart disease. Over time, persistent blood sugar abnormalities may impair nerve function, damage the vision, and lead to a variety of health concerns.

Recognizing Blood Sugar Imbalance Symptoms
Understanding the symptoms of blood sugar imbalance allows you to intervene and take control of your health. Fatigue, mood changes, strong cravings, frequent thirst, increased urination, and difficulty focusing are all common symptoms. By recognizing these indications, you may make educated choices to avoid protracted periods of volatility and regulate your blood sugar levels.

As we get to the end of this chapter, you'll be well-equipped to ride the Sugar Rollercoaster. You may achieve improved energy stability, emotional balance, and long-term health by acknowledging the highs and lows of blood sugar surges and using mindful ways to moderate them.

Chapter 3: Nourishing Your Body

The Influence of Nutrient-Rich Foods

The transformational potential of nutrient-rich meals is at the heart of robust health and balanced blood sugar. Food is more than simply nourishment; it is the basis upon which our well-being is based. This chapter delves into the surprising influence that our dietary choices have on blood sugar regulation and general health, examining how nutrient-rich foods may be our allies in our quest for vitality.

Nutrient-rich foods have a high density of vital nutrients in comparison to their calorie level. Whole grains, colorful veggies, lean meats, healthy fats, and legumes are examples of these foods. When we emphasize nutrient-dense foods, we increase our consumption of vitamins, minerals, fiber, and antioxidants, all of which are important for maintaining healthy blood sugar levels and general metabolic health.

Creating a Well-balanced Diet for Blood Sugar Control

Creating a balanced diet that maintains blood sugar levels is an art form. It necessitates an awareness of the many functions that carbs, proteins, and lipids play in the energy control of our bodies. Here's how to create a blood sugar-controlling food plan:

• Carbohydrates: Choose complex carbs with a low glycemic index (GI). These carbs gradually release glucose, giving prolonged energy without creating sharp surges. Consume whole grains such as quinoa, brown rice, and whole wheat bread. Include colorful veggies that are high in fiber and important nutrients.

• Proteins: Lean proteins are necessary for blood sugar regulation. Include skinless fowl, fish, eggs, tofu, and beans as sources. Protein helps to balance blood sugar by decreasing glucose absorption, keeping you full and energetic.

• Healthy fats include avocados, almonds, and virgin olive oil. These fats not only benefit general health, but they also aid in satiety, lowering the chance of overeating and blood sugar increases.

• Portion Control: Be mindful of portion sizes. Overeating, even with nutrient-dense meals, may result in an excess of calories, which can influence blood sugar levels. Listen to your body's appetite and satiety indicators.

• Balanced Meals: Aim for meals that are well-balanced in terms of carbs, proteins, and healthy fats. This combination helps to balance blood sugar levels, allowing for a more consistent flow of energy.

Practical Guidelines for Mindful Eating

Mindful eating is a powerful discipline that improves blood sugar regulation and builds a deeper connection with our food. Here are some helpful hints for incorporating mindful eating into your everyday routine:

• Slow Down: Take your time eating and savoring each mouthful. This allows your body time to communicate fullness, reducing overeating.

• Engage Your Senses: Pay attention to your food's tastes, textures, and scents. Fully enjoying your meals increases your enjoyment of them.

• Reduce Distractions: Avoid eating in front of devices or while doing other things. To be present in the moment, concentrate exclusively on your food.

• Chew completely: Chewing extensively promotes digestion and enables your body to more easily access nutrients.

• Listen to the signals coming from your body: Acquire the ability to differentiate between genuine hunger and feelings of compulsion. Pay attention to your body's cues and react appropriately.

Blood Sugar Control Tip for the Elderly

Blood sugar management becomes more crucial as we age. Elderly people confront special problems, however, there are certain ways they may use to efficiently regulate blood sugar:

• Maintain Physical exercise: Engage in regular physical exercise, even if it is in tiny quantities. Low-impact workouts such as walking, swimming, and moderate yoga may help increase insulin sensitivity and blood sugar levels.

• Make Fiber a Priority: Include fiber-rich foods in your diet such as whole grains, vegetables, fruits, and legumes. Fiber slows glucose absorption and adds to a sensation of fullness.

• Distribute carbs: Rather than ingesting significant quantities of carbs in a single meal, spread them out equally throughout the day. This method helps to avoid blood sugar increases.

• Hydration: Drink plenty of water. Drinking water may help manage hunger and may improve blood sugar levels.

• Regular Medical Check-ups: It is important to get regular check-ups with healthcare specialists. Blood sugar levels may be affected by medications and medical conditions, and healthcare practitioners can give specific advice.

We've unearthed the art of fueling your body for maximum blood sugar management and general health in this chapter. You go on a path that allows you to create lifelong well-being by embracing nutrient-rich foods, preparing balanced meals, practicing mindful eating, and adjusting tactics for various life phases. The decisions you make now may define a future of vitality, energy, and blood sugar balance.

Chapter 4: Balanced Lifestyle Practices

Lifestyle choices are the threads that bind our general well-being in the complex fabric of blood sugar regulation. Beyond what we put on our plate, our daily activities and decisions are crucial in directing the delicate symphony of blood sugar levels. This chapter explores the substantial impact of consistent physical exercise, stress reduction, and sound sleep on blood sugar homeostasis, highlighting the interdependence of these lifestyle variables and their capacity for transformation.

The Value of Frequently Engaging in Physical Activity

As a maestro guiding a mellow tune of blood sugar management, exercise develops. Regular exercise increases the body's sensitivity to insulin, allowing cells to use glucose for energy more effectively. Exercise and insulin work together dynamically to generate a pattern that lessens the likelihood of unexpected spikes and drops in blood sugar levels.

By improving glucose absorption by muscles, aerobic workouts including brisk walking, running, swimming, and cycling efficiently reduce blood sugar levels.

By boosting muscle development and improving insulin sensitivity, resistance training, which includes exercises like weightlifting and bodyweight routines, contributes.

Consistency is essential for anybody looking to maximize the advantages of exercise for maintaining blood sugar homeostasis. Aim for two days of weight training per week coupled with at least 150 minutes of moderate-intensity aerobic exercise.

Management of Stress and Blood Sugar Effects

Blood sugar levels may be dramatically impacted by stress, the contemporary crescendo that often accompanies our fast-paced existence. The body gets ready for a "fight or flight" reaction when stress hormones like cortisol spike, which causes the liver to release glucose into the circulation. This may eventually lead to increased blood sugar levels in those who are under a lot of stress.

This biological reaction finds a relaxing counterbalance in stress management. Utilizing relaxation methods like yoga, deep breathing, meditation, and mindfulness helps lower cortisol levels and encourage a more stable blood sugar environment.

Stress reduction is also aided by engaging in hobbies, going outside, and building social ties.

The Importance of Good Sleep for Blood Sugar Control

The nightly serenade of sleep is crucial for maintaining a healthy blood sugar level. The delicate balance between insulin and glucose may be upset by sleep deprivation and poor sleep quality, which can result in insulin resistance and increased blood sugar levels.

The body goes through important activities during restorative sleep, including hormone control, immune system bolstering, and tissue repair. Sleep disturbances may cause insulin resistance, a rise in hunger, and weight gain—all of which are connected to blood sugar abnormalities.

Prioritize good sleep hygiene by keeping a regular sleep schedule, establishing a relaxing nighttime ritual, and providing a cozy sleeping environment. To encourage the best possible blood sugar health, aim for 7-9 hours of unbroken sleep each night.

Balancing lifestyle practices for harmony

Lifestyle choices play a significant role in the story of blood sugar regulation since they determine how our health develops over time. We create a symphony that harmonizes blood sugar levels, promotes resilience, and cultivates vitality by participating in regular physical exercise, controlling stress, and placing a priority on sound sleep.

Regular exercise gives us the ability to help our bodies use glucose efficiently, reducing unpredictable variations. We carry out a calming counterbalance via stress management to stop cortisol-induced increases. The gentle coda is good sleep, which promotes insulin sensitivity and maintains general health.

As we go through this chapter, we understand that, like the notes in a song, our lifestyle choices weave a tapestry of balance that reverberates throughout our lives. By adopting these lifestyle practices, we promote blood sugar balance, promote a harmonious relationship with our bodies, and nurture well-being that extends well beyond the domain of numbers and measures.

Chapter 5: Recipes for Change

Food serves as a blank canvas on which blood sugar harmony may be created. In this chapter, we explore the world of transforming recipes and discover how delicious, nutrient-dense meals may support healthy blood sugar levels. We'll explore the sometimes-disregarded relationship between water and blood sugar, as well as clever eating strategies that maintain levels.

Delicious and Filling Meals to Balance Blood Sugar

Consider each meal as a chance to provide your body with a symphony of tastes and nutrients that synchronize to maintain blood sugar stability. Start with breakfast; try a substantial serving of porridge with fresh fruit, nuts, and almond butter on top. Oats provide complex carbs, which when paired with the protein and good fats found in nuts and nut butter reduce increases in blood sugar that happen too quickly.

A bright salad with lush greens, lean protein (such as grilled chicken or chickpeas), and a variety of brilliant veggies might be served for lunch.

This combination promotes a consistent release of glucose, while veggies high in fiber help maintain energy levels.

Consider pairing lean meats, such as salmon or tofu, with healthful grains, like quinoa or brown rice, and roasted veggies for supper. These mixtures provide a wide variety of nutrients that regulate blood sugar and promote general health.

Smart Snacking Strategies to Maintain Your Levels
Between meals, snacking offers a chance to maintain blood sugar equilibrium. Choose complete foods instead, such as a cup of mixed nuts, a serving of hummus-topped carrot sticks, or Greek yogurt with berries. These snacks include protein, good fats, and fiber, which combined help to slow down digestion and avoid unexpected increases in blood sugar.

Consider a piece of fruit with a modest amount of cottage cheese or a slice of whole-grain bread with avocado to stave off afternoon cravings. These options provide a filling combination of protein and carbs, ensuring that your energy level is consistent throughout the day.

Hydration and Blood Sugar: What You Need to Know

The relationship between water and blood sugar is a key but frequently ignored part of a healthy lifestyle. Staying appropriately hydrated enhances the body's capacity to manage blood sugar levels. Water contributes to carrying glucose to cells, where it's utilized for energy. Dehydration may lead to greater quantities of glucose in the circulation.

Make it a habit to drink water consistently throughout the day. Herbal teas, infused water with lemon or cucumber, and water-rich fruits like watermelon and oranges may contribute to your daily hydration requirements while encouraging blood sugar balance.

Incorporating Transformative Recipes

The transforming power of recipes resides in their capacity to convert ordinary items into remarkable experiences that enhance blood sugar balance. Each meal and snack is a time to discover tastes, textures, and combinations that fuel your body and maintain your energy.

Consider making a weekly meal plan that contains a range of nutrient-rich meals, guaranteeing a balanced distribution of carbs, proteins, and healthy fats throughout the day. Experiment with new ingredients and dishes, enjoying the delight of culinary discovery.

Remember that the aim is to build a sustainable strategy. Incorporate the concepts of balanced nutrition into your daily routine, one meal at a time. By leveraging the transforming potential of recipes, you develop a culinary journey that not only thrills your taste senses but also allows you to attain enduring blood sugar balance, vigor, and a revitalized feeling of well-being.

Chapter 6: The Sugar Shift Action Plan

As we begin on the Sugar Shift journey, it's crucial to have a complete action plan that allows us to achieve real, permanent improvements in our health. This chapter exposes the Sugar Shift Action Plan, a blueprint meant to help you through the transformative process of obtaining balanced blood sugar, establishing realistic objectives, measuring progress, making required modifications, and eventually sustaining a lifetime of well-being.

Setting Realistic Goals for Your Health Transformation

Setting clear, realistic objectives is the cornerstone of every effective transition. Whether your emphasis is on stabilizing blood sugar levels, maintaining a healthy weight, or just improving overall well-being, the key is to make your objectives precise, measurable, attainable, relevant, and time-bound (PMART).

For example, a PMART goal may be to limit your daily added sugar consumption to a certain number, such as fewer than 25 grams, during the next three months.

This objective is precise (added sugar consumption), measurable (less than 25 grams), realistic (based on dietary modifications), relevant (supporting blood sugar balance), and time-bound (during the next three months).

It's crucial to remember that change takes time, and improvement may occur in little stages. Celebrate each milestone along the journey, whether it's a drop in blood sugar levels, more energy, or better general well-being. These victories inspire your enthusiasm to continue on the road of the Sugar Shift.

Tracking Your Progress and Making Adjustments
Tracking your success is a critical element of the Sugar Shift Action Plan. Regular monitoring helps you to measure the efficacy of your efforts and make required modifications. Consider maintaining a notebook where you record your meals, physical activity, blood sugar measurements (if appropriate), and any pertinent notes about how you feel. By analyzing this information often, you may spot trends, highlight areas where you're succeeding, and uncover areas that could require development.

If you discover that a certain dietary adjustment or workout plan is not delivering the intended results, be prepared to adapt your strategy.

Flexibility is crucial on this journey since everyone's body reacts differently.

Seek expert support, such as speaking with a qualified dietitian or healthcare specialist, to help understand your progress and make educated choices regarding revisions to your action plan. Remember, the Sugar Shift is about identifying what works best for you and adapting the approach appropriately.

Maintaining Balance for a Lifetime of Wellness

The Sugar Shift isn't a short-term remedy; it's a lifestyle makeover aimed at supporting long-term well-being. As you move along this path, concentrate on creating durable habits that become vital to your everyday life. Embrace the concepts of a balanced diet, mindful eating, regular physical exercise, stress management, and excellent sleep as pillars of your continuing well-being.

Maintaining equilibrium is key. Allow yourself occasional indulgences while keeping conscious of portion sizes and the overall influence on your blood sugar.

 Recognize that life may provide problems and temptations, but your increased knowledge and abilities equip you to negotiate these circumstances with grace.

Consider adding stress-reduction methods, such as meditation or deep breathing, into your daily routine to promote both blood sugar control and general well-being. Prioritize sleep as a critical pillar of health, acknowledging its tremendous effect on your body's capacity to manage blood sugar.

By incorporating these practices into your life, you're developing a firm basis for long-term well-being. The Sugar Shift Action Plan is not a momentary remedy; it's a lifetime commitment to nourishing your health and energy.

Incorporating the Sugar Shift Action Plan

The Sugar Shift Action Plan isn't just a plan; it's a transforming blueprint that enables you to take charge of your health and fitness. By establishing realistic objectives, measuring progress, making changes, and maintaining balance, you're constructing a sustainable road to a lifetime of blood sugar harmony.

As you continue your Sugar Shift journey, bear in mind that each step you take is a step toward enduring well-being.

Celebrate your triumphs, learn from your experiences, and remain dedicated to the ideals that have become a part of your everyday life. By accepting the Sugar Shift Action Plan, you're not simply altering your habits—you're improving your connection with health, one empowered decision at a time.

Conclusion: Embrace the Sweet Change

As we draw the curtain on this transforming trip into the subtleties of blood sugar balance, it's time to reflect on the deep changes you've begun and the hopeful road that lies ahead. This ending chapter is a celebration of your health improvement, a reminder of the continuous road toward balanced blood sugar, and an invitation to be inspired by the tales of individuals who have embraced the Sugar Shift with success.

Celebrating Your Health Transformation

Every stride you've made on the road to blood sugar balance is a testimonial to your devotion to well-being. Celebrate the improvements you've made, both great and little. Recognize the work you've made in learning, adjusting, and making decisions that value your health. Your journey is a reflection of your devotion, resilience, and the power of good transformation.

Pause to appreciate the changes you've seen — whether it's greater energy, stable emotions, weight control, or better general health. Each success is a milestone on your journey to enduring well-being.

The Ongoing Journey to Balanced Blood Sugar

Embracing healthy blood sugar isn't a destination; it's a lifetime process. As you go ahead, remember that health is not characterized by perfection, but by consistency and dedication. Continue to practice the ideas you've learned – from selecting nutrient-rich meals to participating in regular physical exercise and developing mindfulness.

Stay alert to your body's cues, assess your progress, and make modifications as appropriate. Life is full of twists and turns, and your approach to blood sugar control should be adaptive to changing situations. Embrace obstacles as chances to learn and develop, and consider failures as stepping stones toward greater resilience.

Inspiring Stories of Sugar Shift Success

Drawing inspiration from those who have launched on the Sugar Shift journey may fuel your drive and create a feeling of camaraderie. Read accounts of people who have experienced exceptional achievement in obtaining balanced blood sugar. Their examples underline the transformational power of devotion and give insights into techniques that have proved beneficial.

These success stories remind us that the Sugar Shift is feasible, regardless of age, background, or circumstances. They reveal the possibilities that lie when you commit to your health and well-being.

Embrace the Sweet Change

As you embark on this new chapter of your life, appreciate the beautiful transformation you've started. Remember that your health is a priceless treasure, and your decisions can determine your vitality and quality of life. The road toward balanced blood sugar is a journey toward empowerment, resilience, and a future loaded with possibilities.

Celebrate every milestone, accept the trials, and relish the progress you make. The Sugar Shift is more than a notion — it's a lifestyle, a philosophy, and a road to well-being. With the information you've received and the dedication you've shown, you're able to manage the difficulties of blood sugar balance with elegance and poise.

Embrace the pleasant shift, and take it ahead with you as you develop a life distinguished by vigor, well-being, and the promise of enduring health.

Your journey has just started, and the road ahead is lined with the promise of a future rich with health and the delight of experiencing life to the fullest.